THIS BOOK

BELONGS TO

....

....

Thank you for Purchasing my book and taking the time to read it from front to back. I am always grateful when a reader chooses my work and I hope you enjoyed it!

With the vast selection available online, I am touched that you chose to be purchasing my work and take valuable time out of your life to read it. My hope is that you feel you made the right decision.

I very much would like to know what you thought of the book. Please take the time to write an honest and informative review on Amazon.com. Your experience and opinions will be of great benefit to me and those readers looking to make an informed choice.

With much thanks.

Table of Contents

Introduction

CBD is one of the most controversial topics these days. Over the years, debates have been waged among experts on the efficacy of CBD in treating certain illnesses. Some sectors oppose the use of it while some sectors promote it.

To prove the claim that it is effective in treating certain illnesses, experiments and studies were done and are continuously being done. To this day, a lot of clinical studies yielded positive results proving the efficacy of CBD. One of the clinical studies which you will be able to read in this book has been the key to unlock the FDA's apprehension in using CBD to treat epileptic seizures. Yes, you've read it correctly; there is one CBD-based medical drug that is now being used.

Despite the positive results of the many clinical studies, there are still gray areas to cover. Some studies, while being regarded as successful, lack precision and direction on how CBD will treat a particular disease. However, this does not mean that the doors are closed. This only shows the need for more clinical studies until that 'Aha! Moment' has been discovered.

Abuse and addiction is another critical item that's bothering the minds of the authorities and medical professionals. Strict guidelines should not only be focused on regulating the use of CBD but stricter guidelines in sourcing the supply which is the cannabis plant. Added to that is the control measures in the production and distribution so that abuse and addiction will not contribute to socio-economic problems.

This book will take you on a tour of CBD. The what, why, where, when, and how of CBD will be explained simply. At the end of your reading, you will have all the basic knowledge about CBD. If you are interested in exploring CBD, then this book is for you.

Chapter 1

CBD (Cannabinoid) Explained

CBD is one of the components of the plant Cannabis. There are two broad classifications of Cannabis types that contain a considerable amount of CBD. These are Hemp and Marijuana. Besides CBD, Hemp contains less than 0.3% THC, while Marijuana contains more than 0.3% THC (Tetrahydrocannabinol). Which one is more effective is still being debated.

Here are some facts about Hemp and Marijuana:

Hemp

Hemp became more popular because CBD made from Hemp is legal to consume in all 50 states in the United States since it has a very minimal component of THC (less than 0.03%). The government classifies Hemp as any plant of the Cannabis family that contains less than 0.3% THC.

To create a product for consumption, there are industrial procedures. There are many interventions from extraction to the formulation to delivery to the patient or consumer. These processes depend on who is doing it and how it is done. Despite its popularity, there were claims that patients' conditions were aggravated. This happened due to the presence of other chemical components that were not controlled.

Marijuana

THC is present in Marijuana as well as CBD. CBD is responsible for the therapeutic function while THC has the psychoactive effect or the one that causes that "high feeling" when taken. This is the reason why some have patients are apprehensive about using this CBD type.

Some are claiming that efficacy is at its best when a considerable amount of THC is mixed with CBD.

Israel is one country where the study of Cannabis is allowed and during the studies, hundreds of compounds within the plant have been discovered and 80% are cannabinoids. It has also been discovered that, when mixed, CBD and THC are at their best performance in treating illnesses, such as epilepsy, chronic pain, and insomnia.

In terms of consumption, there is what is called whole plant medicine where the plant is naturally administered. This type is offered by holistic and alternative medicine communities. Another way is fractioned medicine where a synthetic process is used by pharmaceutical companies that have produced a drug, oil, spray, and food additive.

Nonetheless, whether it's hemp or marijuana, it's the presence of CBD that is important. CBD synergizes well with the body systems and has a therapeutic reaction when administered to a patient.

Caution must be observed though because there are manufacturers who are taking advantage of the situation. Since there is a limited source of CBD, they are mixing it with other substances just to make the composition complete for consumption. The target result will still be evident but can no longer be maximized because of the other substances that have been added. A worst case is that the body may react negatively and aggravate the illness being treated. That is why patients need to be careful where they get their CBD supplies. They need to make sure that they get it from trusted sources, the ones recommended by the experts.

"My life has changed thanks to CBD

This is just short of a miracle for me and my wife. I was skeptical at first but my wife insisted because we couldn't get her regular medicine for anxiety due to insurance problems living in the US. I ate one 10mg gummy cause what the hay I paid for them. Almost immediate relief from my aches and pains. I felt better than I had in months. And the effects even carried over to the next night at work where I was literally kicking my heels and singing I felt great! I can't imagine how much relief it's brought my wife. Just wanted to testify. Rock on world." – Reddit member

Chapter 2

Debunking the Misconception about CBD

Misconceptions about CBD are understandable. This is because people are still debating on its efficacy and experts are still exploring the perfect mixture and components that will not prove harmful when administered to humans. Here are 10 of the most common misconceptions.

However, this is not to convince you that CBD is for you. This is just to set the record straight.

"My friend told me that Hemp and Marijuana are the same."

There are two broad classifications of Cannabis types that contain a considerable amount of CBD. What's confusing people about them is both of them have a considerable amount of CBD. While this is true, Marijuana has a THC component while Hemp has less than 0.3%. THC produces that "high feeling" effect when ingested thus making Marijuana prohibited in most parts of the country.

"It's under Schedule 1 status; we cannot test or do experiments."
The federal government marked Cannabis under Schedule 1 status and thus institutions are very cautious in doing their experiments as they might be breaking the law. However, Columbia University braved the way by testing CBD in treating Glioblastoma. This is the most common brain tumor in humans. As CBD was administered to a patient, the death of cancer cells began to take place without damaging the healthy cells. Israel, the UK, Italy, and Brazil are other countries conducting constant and aggressive research on CBD.

"It was not effective when I tried it."

CBD is not first aid. It is also not a pain reliever. What it does is treat chronic pain and not acute pain. What does this mean?

First, ask yourself if your symptoms are something the CBD can alleviate. Next, experiments for its good effects were done in periods. So stop thinking that it will eliminate the symptoms immediately after taking it. It may, but also you may need some time to feel its effect.

"I can use it wherever and whenever I want because it is 100% legal."

This depends on where you're residing. Many parts of the world still do not have acceptance for these two substances. The use is being prevented with the notion that these two substances result in addiction.

Hemp Farming was legalized in 2018. Hemp is composed of CBD but is not addictive. So all hemp-derived products are legal to sell and consume. However, strict caution reminds consumers to purchase from trusted sources only. This is to ensure that no other components were mixed with the hemp-derived product that may cause illness to be aggravated.

"There's no scientific proof that CBD cures."

In the summer of 2018, the FDA approved the use of Epidiolex. This is a CBD-based drug that helps manage epileptic seizure disorders.

Yes, there are still many who are apprehensive of this claim but facts are present to prove it. Continuous studies are being done to intensify the claim that CBD can treat more illnesses.

"I don't want to undergo a drug test because I will test positive with addictive compounds."

It again depends on the kind of drug test being conducted. If the drug test wants to know the level of CBD in your body while you are under CBD administration, it will show positive results. But when it comes to drug testing, it is the traces of THC that is being tested. THC is the culprit because it results in addictive behavior. Full Spectrum CBD products contain less than 0.3% THC and when using them you may test positive on a drug test. There are Broad Spectrum and Isolate products that do not have any trace of THC so when using them the test will be negative.

"CBD will make me high."

Again this is a clear misconception. CBD will not make you high - THC will. If you're consuming Hemp you will never experience a euphoric feeling. But if you using marijuana-derived products, there is a high probability that you will feel high. It depends on the level of THC present in what you've taken.

"CBD alone will not heal me so what I need is Marijuana."

CBD is effective on its own. It will still provide a therapeutic effect for some distressing symptoms. The reason for this misconception is because of what they call the entourage effect, where CBD will be more effective when mixed with other cannabis compounds like THC, and this mixture will elevate its efficacy to treat illness.

"I need a higher dosage so I will be healed faster."

This is something relative and never an absolute claim. It always depends on the patient taking it. Experts, however, highly advise that slow progress is better thus low doses are needed. There are other factors to consider when taking CBD, such as metabolism, underlying illness, body weight, activities being done, and even demographics. All these must be considered before deciding the amount of CBD that is right for a patient.

"CBD is just a scam and they can get more money from it."

Since the introduction of CBD to the market, ideas were developed as to how to further boost its use to help those in need. Some ideas were to include it in small amounts to the food eaten or formulate it together with oils, or sprays. On this premise, the price of their product will be a bit higher than usual.

Maybe a governing body must make laws for these measures to control the use of CBD with other commercial products.

Though all of these misconceptions have been debunked, nothing compares to doing your research and study. If you are serious about considering CBD, you must use the right perspective. Don't take it half-hearted. Make sure that when you take it, your brain aligns. It's like believing that after you take paracetamol your headache will be gone. The medicine will do the therapeutic role and your brain will do the psychological cure.

"I have Lupus and was MISERABLE! The aches and pains were awful and the medication they gave me rarely made the pain vanish but did make me puke and my stomach cramp! (FUN TIMES!) Finally, I started with CBD and I can get through the day without being sick and miserable. I am so grateful to have finally listened to my friend who kept urging me to try CBD." – Reddit member

Chapter 3

Chemical and Physical Component of CBD

This chapter will give you a deeper understanding of CBD. Chemical components will be discussed to better understand where it is derived and its curative effects.

The plant Cannabis has over 400 components and around 60 are Cannabinoids. This is to highlight that Cannabis is not concentrated with CBD or THC alone even if they are the most known cannabinoids. The 60+ cannabinoids present in the plant are grouped into subclasses:

• Cannabidiols (CBD)
• Tetrahydrocannabinols (THC)
• Cannabichromenes (CBC)
• Cannabinol (CBN) and cannabinodiol (CBDL)
• Cannabigerols (CBG)
• Other cannabinoids (such as cannabicyclol (CBL), cannabielsoin (CBE), cannabidiol (CBT) and other miscellaneous types).

These cannabinoids are differentiated by the extent of its psychological impact. CBN, CBG, and CBC do not contain such effect while THC, CBN, CBDL possess it in varying degrees.

Among these, CBD is the most extracted component since it has the curative part of Cannabis. It also occupies 40% of the Cannabinoids resin extracted from Cannabis. Next to it is the THC, which even if it has a psychoactive effect, many believe that when it is combined with CBD, the curative effect works best. However, there is only a certain percentage of THC allowed to be mixed to CBD to avoid the psychoactive effect to happen because it has the highest amount of psychoactive components among the Cannabinoids. Over time, the Cannabis plant if left unused, the THC in it transforms into CBN which is less psychologically active than THC hence, decreasing the psychoactive effect on the brain.

CBD is insoluble in water but soluble to other organic compounds. It crystallizes into a colorless solid under room temperature. In alkaline or basic environment, it is transformed into quinone which is a known oxidizing agent. In an acidic environment, it reacts with THC. CBD has a molecular weight of 314.5 g/mol.

Cannabinoids have receptors called CB1, also called anandamide. It binds with CB2 and when they bind, the process is called an endogenous cannabinoid system. These two receptors interact with specific receptors located in the central nervous system. The reaction is strong in the limbic and mesolimbic systems of the brain. The limbic system is the one responsible for the memory, psychomotor activities, and cognition activities of the brain. The mesolimbic system is related to feelings and pain perceptions. Not only that, but CBD also has receptors to interact with the cardiovascular system. It reacts with the adenosine receptor and enhances the release of dopamine, which is also associated with feelings. This explains why CBD is said to cure chronic pain, strong seizures, anxiety, and a lot more that is related to the limbic and mesolimbic systems in the brain.

Studies have stated that it is the THC that plays a major part in activating the CB1 and CB2 receptors thus, the dangers of creating a strong psychoactive effect. The good news is that it is antagonized by CBD. CBD has the role of blocking the THC effects when it activates CB1 and CB2 receptors. However, since CBD has multiple mechanisms, there will be times where instead of being an antagonist of the psychoactive effect, it may enhance it.

"For the story, I gave CBD oil to my mom a few month ago, and the day after she told me "I don't know if it is the CBD but I haven't slept that good in years".

So I was really happy to see that I had an answer for one of her issue." – Reddit member

Chapter 4

Forms of CBD

Due to its popularity because of proven positive effects, the demand for CBD has increased too. Many want to try this product with high hopes of curing a long-term illness that no medicine or procedure has been able to address. CBD is legal but only to some extent. The legalities depend on where you are located.

The hard truth is not everyone has direct access to CBD. The process of acquiring, formulating, and marketing is so complex that it is very difficult to have easy access to it. There may be 'under the table' selling but the product will not have come from a trusted source and may just aggravate your condition instead of alleviating it.

It is important to understand the different forms of CBD so you can find out which one is best suited for you. Each form contains different levels of CBD concentration. The effect may be direct or indirect depending on how you consume it. The part that is being treated may be systemic or localized depending on the form you are using.

CBD Lotion/Cream/Balm/Roll-on/Salves

This form targets topically. The effect is localized depending on the area where it is applied. CBD in this form is usually mixed with menthol and essential oils with mint and mild flower extract. This is used to relieve muscle and joint pain, any part of the body that is swelling, and even arthritis. The effect can be felt within hours. You can reapply this as needed.

This can also be used to treat eczema and psoriasis. When applied to the affected area, the effect can be felt within 15 minutes.

CBD Vape

This is by far the most popular form used. This is due to the high bioavailability effect which allows an almost instant effect when inhaled. When inhaled, the product goes directly to the lungs and then is distributed through the bloodstream. The effect, after inhaling, lasts from 90 minutes to 3 hours.

CBD Oil/Tinctures

Tinctures are alcohol-based. Since it has been proven that oil is absorbed easily by the body, oil is now being infused with CBD. To apply it, a drop is taken under the tongue. The tongue is composed of many tiny capillaries or tiny nerves that will transport CBD through the body. Based on a study, this is more effective than taking it orally. When CBD is taken orally, it is processed in the gastrointestinal tract where the process of absorption and distribution is slower.

The relief will be felt within 20 minutes and will last up to 8 hours. There is no specific dosage for this form. You can take as much or as little as you want. CBD oil, by the way, is also sometimes included in baked products.

CBD Spray

CBD Spray is used to treat localized issues, such as skin problems like eczema and psoriasis. This can also treat burns, rashes, and other skin irritations by spraying it on the affected areas.

CBD Capsule

If the desire is to have systemic relief, the CBD capsule is highly recommended. There's nothing to worry about the dosage as it is already set in the capsule. However, there is low bioavailability in CBD capsules since it is taken into the digestive tract, undergoes metabolism, and some of the contents are filtered out during the digestion. However, if you're on-the-go or traveling, this is the most convenient form. It also gives long-lasting relief which may last for several hours.

CBD Edibles

Gummy bear is the most common form of CBD edibles. A gummy is usually composed of 5 milligrams of CBD. This is also popular because of its sweet taste. Just like the CBD capsule, this is good for people on-the-go. It has the same impact as the CBD capsule.

Other forms of CBD edibles are chocolates, infused water, smoothies, and powders.

CBD Bath Salts

Over time, CBD forms have evolved. CBD is now also infused into bath salts. Anyone using it normally feels a calming effect. Note that the calming effect is different from the psychoactive effect so there's no worry about using it.

"Been taking CBD for about a month now (anxiety). Started it with flowers but am now doing the tincture.

Besides feeling anxiety free (keep in mind my anxiety isn't severe and I can manage it without meds) I am shocked at how much more energy I'm having and even though the flower made me a bit sleepy, I was still way more productive than usual. For example, two ballet classes per week is all I could manage but I am now taking 5 classes per week.

Should have started it months ago" – Reddit member

Chapter 5

<u>Why Use CBD Over Other Medicine</u>

There are no known advantages of CBD over medicines except for these three major reasons:

It is natural since it comes from a plant

CBD is an extract of the Cannabis plant, hence a natural treatment. It is unlike other drugs that are synthetic and made of different chemical components. The impact of ingesting chemicals may not be felt immediately, but over time it will be felt by your body. When a person needs to medicate regularly and the medication is in a form of capsule or tablet that is composed of chemicals and other synthetic ingredients, the doctor will also give the patient a vitamin for the liver. Since the liver acts as an absorbent or filter, it is highly affected when a chemical compound is ingested by the body. The sad part here is even the medication for the liver is chemically produced.

With CBD, we are assured of its purest form. Extraction and transformation are done naturally. It will be mixed with other forms such as oil, but natural ingredients are used.

The effect can be felt right away because it targets the bloodstreams

Most of the drugs that we ingest are in the form of a capsule or tablets. Since it is swallowed, these drugs will go through our digestive system. Digestion is one of the longest processes in our body. As such, the effect of the medication will not be felt immediately.

Inducing any medication directly into the bloodstream gives an almost immediate effect. The cure can be instant. The best CBD form for this is the CBD oil.

There is also a tendency for the medicine to lose its efficiency when it interacts with other substances in the digestive system. Losing its efficiency means you need to intake more of it to optimize the effect.

Mixes well with other forms

CBD mixes well with other forms of the substance. There are many ways to take CBD. This gives CBD an advantage over the conventional capsule, syrup, or tablet. In its form, you can easily detect the level of CBD.

This also provides authorized distributors with more options to sell their products. As of this writing, continuous studies are being done to discover other forms that can mix well with CBD.

This is not to replace the conventional medication that your doctors prescribe. This is just for information that CBD could be advantageous over the usual medicines. Perhaps a paracetamol tablet can be replaced by a drop of CBD oil. They are different in forms but the latter provides a faster result. You choose. As long as it is approved by your doctor, there's nothing to worry about.

"Never had any experience or expectations basically assumed it was a placebo effect. I can only extol the positives. Just a feeling of calm. My mind always races from one thought to the next but the CBD definitely quieted that. No loss of motivation and definitely not high. Just calm. As a 56 year old middle class married Midwest male I'm throwing my hat in for complete legalization. I was never against but I'm definitely pro." – Reddit member

Chapter 6

Dangers of CBD

Much has been said about the benefits of CBD. However, it is also critical to know its dangers. No one ever said that it is very safe to use. Everything is still blurry and that's why continuous studies are being done. Here are some of the dangers. These are based on studies and experiments conducted.

May Increase Liver Toxicity

While CBD is made from a natural ingredient which is the Cannabis plant, it reacts with an enzyme called cytochrome P450 complex. This enzyme is disrupted when it interacts with CBD. When this enzyme is disrupted, it impacts the liver's ability to break down toxins.

Effects when Treating Epilepsy

FDA approved the commercial use of the CBD drug called Epidiolex due to its proven effectiveness. However, there is an adverse reaction in the body causing the patient to have the following reactions:

- Lethargy
- Loss of Appetite
- Problems in Urinating
- Difficulty in Breathing
- Gastrointestinal Problems
- Infections
- Allergic Reactions and Rashes
- Liver Problems

Can be Addictive

CBD in its purest form doesn't contain any psychoactive component that leads to addiction. However, since it impacts the central nervous system, there may be effects leading to addiction. This is not absolute but is relative to the patient's reaction. A person using CBD must be strictly observed.

Leads to Depression and Suicidal Thoughts

This reaction is caused by CBD interacting directly with the receptors in the central nervous system. This is relative to the patient's reaction. These symptoms are something that should not be taken for granted. A person with prolonged use of CBD must be interviewed from time to time to detect the presence of these effects.

Interaction with other Medicines Poses Danger

Interaction of two or more drugs when taken at the same time is common. However, the effect varies. Some interactions can pose dangers, much like CBD interacting with other medicines. This is mainly caused by CBD's ability to disrupt the liver enzyme called cytochrome P450 complex. As it disrupts that enzyme, it also disrupts the liver to function well. A liver that is not functioning properly will not be able to metabolize other drugs taken, hence disrupting its curative effects.

Another risk to the liver is the interaction itself. Having too much to metabolize overtaxes the liver. This will lead to its inability to function as expected.

With all these dangers considered, it is safe to say that CBD is not 100% safe to use. Perhaps this is the reason why legalities are still a big controversy in some parts of the world. CBD itself is safe, but when it interacts with other substances, there is risk. If you still want to use CBD or as prescribed by your doctor, you just need to be cautious and observant of the symptoms you are feeling after taking CBD. A regular visit to your doctor will make everything safe. Don't wait for all the symptoms to happen. Don't wait for the symptoms to be an illness. Immediately consult your doctor.

"As a former pot head, I had placed the whole CBD thing into the same category as healing crystals, essential oils, voodoo and other such nonsense.

I am 44 and have had sleeping problems my entire life. Recently I decided to say F it and give it a shot.

I am now going for my 5th night. I use an oura ring for sleep tracking and recovery. All of my sleep numbers and exerciser recovery has done thru the roof. My resting heart rate has dropped 5 beats, my HRV has doubled. I can't believe it. It's like a miracle." – Reddit member

Chapter 7

Administering CBD

How to Administer CBD

The answer to this depends on the type of CBD you purchase. The ideal is you must know the suitable CBD for your condition before you make a purchase. People's reactions to CBD vary. It's not a 'one-size fits all'. You must not rely on others' reactions to the substance or actual experience if you're still deciding whether to take it or not.

Since it is widely accepted by many medical practitioners, you can always seek their advice about using it to treat an illness. However, if you are like many who just use CBD topically to ease pain, swelling, or even itchiness, you can directly buy the specific form suited for those symptoms from many over-the-counter retailers.

Each form and type of CBD is unique and depends on a lot of factors. It is not a good idea to take CBD randomly just because you want to know if it will relieve your symptoms or not. You need to consider two important factors:

- Choosing the CBD that fits your body and lifestyle

- Identifying the right dosage that will relieve your condition

One thing for sure, CBD has multiple mechanisms. If you self-medicate, it may not provide the relief you need. When this happens, you've wasted not just money but the opportunity of CBD to prove its curative claims. That is why it is important that you take the time to decide how you will use CBD. Below are the methods of administering CBD.

Applied Directly to the Skin

This is called topical application and there are certain CBD forms for this kind of application. Most of the cases being treated by topical applications are skin problems, such as eczema, allergies, and skin asthma. Topical application is also used to treat body aches or localized pain. It could be used to relieve your muscle and joint aches or used to massage to soothe nerve endings and increase blood circulation.

With topical application, the result is almost instant and lasts for a few hours. You might need to apply more and more frequently until you feel the results. Most CBD of this type is mixed with other ingredients like menthol and these ingredients intensify the therapeutic benefits of CBD.

Edibles

Edibles are the most common way of taking CBD. Tablets and capsules are handy and do not require much effort. Edibles include the information on how much CBD is in one tablet. Usually the amount is presented in milligrams.

The effect may not be felt immediately. This is because the edible still needs to undergo the digestion process which takes time. A person will not be able to ingest 100% of what is taken; only 20%-30% will enter your bloodstream. This is due to the metabolism that transpired during digestion.

Sublingual

This manner of application is done by dropping or spraying a small amount under the tongue where tiny nerves have a direct connection to the sensors of the brain. The result is felt faster compared to taking edibles.

Through Smoking

The popular way of smoking CBD is through vaping and the CBD is inhaled. Since smoke goes into the bloodstream directly, the effect is direct too. You will feel results even after 10 minutes of vaping.

A word of caution: you are exposed to carcinogens when smoking or vaping. So please think twice before choosing this option.

"Wow. I have suffered from paranoia, anxiety and panic attacks for years. I constantly think I'm going insane, feel the need to look behind me when walking on the street, constantly doubting my own thoughts and feelings. When I'm alone at night I can't sleep well because I am scared someone is going to break into my home.

Three days ago I started taking raw CBD oil. All of it is just gone. I don't have those "what if?" -thoughts. I feel calm. I feel safe. It's weird. I am still not sure if the effect is real or just placebo. But I love it. I hope it will continue to work." – Reddit member

Chapter 8

CBD Dosages

Before you get excited about the many benefits that CBD offers make sure you are well acquainted with the dosage that you anticipate taking. Of course, the best thing to do is to sit down with your doctor and have a discussion. CBD is highly sensitive and the effects are not light especially when abused. There is a need to follow very strict guidelines so you are not compromised.

There are five things to consider when determining the dosage of the CBD that will help you feel better. These considerations are body weight, age, physical condition, body chemistry, and most of all, the concentration of CBD in a product.

Dosage can be as small as 20 mg or as large as 1500 mg. When consulting a doctor, consider their words final. You need to follow the directions for whatever is prescribed for you. If there's no recommended dosage, you can start with 20 mg and then increase the dosage by 5 mg as needed.

CBD Dosage Chart

The general rule is to take 1 to 6 mg per 10 lbs. of weight. Here is a sample chart:

Body Weight	Low (Starting) Dose	Medium Dose	High Dose
100 lbs	10-20 mg	21-49 mg	50-60 mg
110 lbs	11-22 mg	23-54 mg	55-66 mg
120 lbs	12-24 mg	25-59 mg	60-72 mg
130 lbs	13-26 mg	27-64 mg	65-78

			mg
140 lbs	14-28 mg	29-69 mg	70-84 mg
150 lbs	15-30 mg	31-74 mg	75-90 mg
160 lbs	16-32 mg	33-79 mg	80-96 mg
170 lbs	17-34 mg	35-84 mg	85-102 mg
180 lbs	18-36 mg	37-89 mg	90-108 mg

As mentioned, this is just a general rule. Depending on the severity of your condition, your daily dose could be higher or lower. What is important is that you don't overdose. It is easier to take less than the required and then just add dosage slowly than taking a huge amount upfront, which may pose a grave problem to your health. You also need to be observant of the after-effects, such as diarrhea, headache, allergies, and other symptoms. Stop using if you have these symptoms.

CBD Dosage per CBD Type

CBD Edibles

These are usually in the form of a capsule or tablet. The recommended CBD dosage will be based on the weight of the patient. Here is the guide:

• Up to 10 mg – Less than 50 lbs.
• 10 mg to 20 mg – 51 to 100 lbs.
• 15 mg to 30 mg - 151 to 200 lbs.
• 20 mg to 50mg – Over 200 lbs.

CBD Vape

One thing that must be taken into consideration for vaping is that the recommended dosage is calculated per day, not per vape. Here's the CBD dosage chart for vapes:

• 15 ml bottle of vape oil with 150 mg CBD is equivalent to 10 mg of CBD per 1 ml dropper
• 15 ml bottle of vape oil with 250 mg CBD is equivalent to 16.66 mg of CBD per 1 ml dropper
• 5 ml bottle of vape oil with 500 mg CBD is equivalent to 100 mg of CBD per 1 ml dropper

Although it is easier to prepare CBD in a vape, this may pose a danger to those who will be able to inhale your vape. You must not do your CBD vaping unless you're alone.

CBD Oil/Tincture

This is, by far, the fastest way to treat an acute attack of any brain problem. A patient uses this type of CBD to immediately treat epileptic seizures. To determine the dosage, you need to know the CBD concentration in the bottle. Per ml, the range of CBD concentration is 100mg to 5000 mg and with that range, the dosage also ranges from 3.3 mg to 166.67 mg.

CBD Lotion

Monitoring dosages in CBD lotions is difficult. A typical bottle of CBD lotion has a concentration of 250 mg to 1500 mg. The dosage cannot be exact because the amount you put on your skin will vary.

Some words of caution: these dosages are general. Visiting a medical expert is highly recommended before you follow these recommendations. You also need to observe the onset of effect after administering it. Observe the effects over 2-3 days to make sure there are no pressing issues.

When is the Best Time to Take CBD?

Those taking CBD want to have its optimal effect and it is important to know the best time of the day to use CBD. The fact is there's no best time. There's no particular formula or recommendation as to when CBD should be administered. It all depends on varying factors such as activities done in a day, metabolism speed, and many more.

At the start of CBD use, the body will adjust to the new substance. Consider observing the effects for a week or two before deciding when the best time for you to take CBD.

Here are some insights to help with your decision-making.

• The effect of CBD Vape is instant. That is why vaping is recommended on an as-needed basis.

• Edibles take effect 30 to 60 minutes after intake. This type of administration is usually done with a meal. If your purpose for taking CBD edibles is to treat insomnia, obviously it is not recommended to take this during breakfast or before going to work.

• Oils/tinctures are like vape and have a fast effect: You will feel the effect 20 minutes after dropping the oil under the tongue.

It depends on what you are treating, on the activities you will do after administering, and the adverse effect it has on your body. It is important to observe your body reactions. You'll discover what time of the day is best to take your CBD dose.

"For the past few years, I've had some issues with letting some bad memories from high school cause self harm, regret, and you could almost say depression. Now with CBD, I don't have those feelings at all. Any time I think about those thoughts now, they have almost no effect on me at all. I swear I haven't felt like this in a while. I remember that even during times when I should be enjoying my hobbies, those memories from high school just keep haunting me, so I can't have as much fun as I should. This is a life saver, and I'm not going to give it up any time soon" – Reddit member

Chapter 9

CBD Buying Guide

CBD can be purchased over the counter and is very easy to acquire. There is a need for scrutiny of the product before deciding to buy to ensure safety. Here are some buying guides that you can consider.

Types of CBD Extract

You need to know what kind of CBD extract is in the product. You may ask your doctor what type of extract would be suited for you. Note that each cannabinoid has its own uses and effects. Here are the types of extract:

• Full Spectrum - this is an extraction of all cannabinoids, including THC and CBD
• Broad Spectrum - this is full spectrum minus THC
• CBD Isolate - Pure CBD only

Manner of CBD Extraction

Read the label. It will tell you if the CBD was extracted via CO2 or Ethanol. Using CO2 preserves the CBD concentration, hence, prevents loss of content which may affect the concentration and dosage when administered. The goal is not to lose concentration. This method requires very expensive equipment which is normally found in professional laboratories. Ethanol extraction involves introducing the solvent ethanol to the hemp plant in order to extract the cannabinoids. What makes one method better comes down to what is the desired end product.

CBD Concentration

Read the label. You should know the CBD concentration you need and then look for it on the labels. Concentration is different from dosages so you must carefully read and understand the labels. When in doubt, ask for assistance.

THC Content

The THC content is critical. THC is what causes a psychoactive effect which is addictive. Abuse will only happen if there is too much THC in the product. The correct amount of THC should not be more than 0.3% of the total solution.

How the Cannabis was grown

You need to buy only US-grown Cannabis because it has passed the agricultural tests required by law for Cannabis. You will be assured of less risk of getting products that were grown using pesticides or other chemicals. According to studies, cannabis grown in Colorado is one of the best in the US.

Other Ingredients in the Product

CBD is mixed with other ingredients to enhance its taste or even effect. Check the ingredients and research the effect of the ingredients when mixed with CBD. You never know what reaction your body will have after ingesting these ingredients. So it's better to be safe than sorry.

Passed Third-Party Laboratory Testing

Any company can claim that their product has been tested and passed all the tests. To be sure of the claims, search for the statistics and the results. Read the labels. If you are still not sure, call the company and ask for the lab test results.

From a Reliable Company

It's fair to say that only large, reputable companies can afford to manufacture quality CBD.

Price

CBD is a bit pricey but in every product, there is always a price ceiling. The cost of CBD per milligram across the industry is around $0.05/milligram (low end) and $0.25/milligram (high end).

Customer Reviews

Customer reviews will help you decide if the product you are about to buy works. However, a universal effect is not guaranteed. The effect of the product for you may differ from what others experienced. Just consider this factor as a guide but must not be the sole deciding factor.

"No anxiety, no nausea (I normally am constantly nauseous from IBS), no anger, so sadness, just happiness and mindfulness. But also no laziness! I'm normally a huge procrastinator but I am getting all of my work done proactively for some reason now. It's really amazing." – Reddit member

Chapter 10

Major Uses of CBD

As discussed in the previous chapters, cannabinoids have an affinity with the receptors in the brain. This is the main reason why cannabinoids can help alleviate symptoms and illness that is centered in the nervous system.

CBD, in particular, has a slightly lower affinity with the brain receptors. It is THC that has a higher affinity thereby causing a psychoactive effect. CBD interacts more with receptors such as an opioid that is responsible for pain management. Another receptor where CBD has stronger affinity is the glycerin receptor that is related to the feel-good hormone serotonin. This is the reason why CBD is good for pain management, anxiety, depression, and other emotional symptoms.

Here are some proven health benefits of CBD:

Regulate Cholesterol and Lower the Risk of Heart Problems

There are two types of cholesterol in our bodies. The good cholesterol is called HDL and the bad cholesterol is called LDL. A high amount of LDL in the body is what causes heart ailments, one of which is a condition called atherosclerosis. In this condition, the heart develops a thicker lining of LDL in the wall of the arteries. This is aggravated by high blood pressure, increased amino acid, and even the presence of infectious microbes in the arteries of the heart. This results in the hardening of the arteries impeding the blood flow throughout the body.

In 2003, 4,000+ participants were observed. The study showed that CBD users had higher HDL content that LDL. In 2005, another experiment was conducted on animals. The subjects were given a low dosage of CBD. The experiment resulted in findings such as a slow progression of atherosclerosis. This experiment was again conducted in 2007 and it proved that CBD has a cardio-protective property.

Boost Brain Health

CBD has neuroprotective properties. This means that CBD helps to manage the health of the brain by removing damaged cells. It also boosts the efficiency of the mitochondria that is responsible for the production of energy in the brain cells.

CBD also reduces glutamate in the brain. Excess glutamate in the brain fires up the stimulation in the brain cells. Overstimulation leads to brain cell damage and even cell death. The introduction of CBD will ease these effects and even provide an anti-inflammatory effect.

Aging has a critical effect on the brain. As we age, the production of new neurons in the brain slows down. This results in the onset of degenerative diseases like neuropathy and Alzheimer's disease. When CBD with a small amount of THC-like substance was introduced, the neuron production increased preventing these harmful effects.

Skin-Friendly

When CBD oil is introduced to the body like lotion, oil, or salve, the CB2 receptors are activated. Thus, the CBD oil can now act to help repair damaged cells due to free radicals from UV rays and other harmful environmental factors. CBD interacts with receptors that are related to oil production in the sebaceous gland. When these interact, healing occurs. Some of the skin issues that can be addressed are acne and psoriasis.

To prove this, a man named Rick Simpson was able to recover from basal cell carcinoma by introducing CBD oil to his skin. This led him to share this information by creating his line of CBD-based products.

CBD lotion is safe because CBD applied topically will not create a psychoactive effect.

Stress Reliever

Taking oral CBD is proven to be effective in managing anxiety. This is related to the activities happening in the limbic and paralimbic portion of the brain. Many studies have proven oral CBD to be effective.

CBD is most effective in relaxing social anxiety. Experiments from previous years have proved this. Subjects were given doses of CBD capsule a few hours before their speaking engagement. These subjects had a public speaking anxiety disorder. After taking CBD, they did not experience an anxiety attack before or during their public speaking address.

A word of caution: You need advice from a medical expert before you take CBD edibles to relax your anxiety disorder. There's a tendency to overdose or to become overly dependent.

Pain Management

There are two types of pain: neuropathic pain, also called chronic pain; and nociceptive pain, also called time-bound pain. Pain is considered chronic if felt 100 days in a year. Experiments and studies have proved that the introduction of CBD in treating pain has managed to ease chronic pain and some cases of nociceptive pain.

The truth is the use of CBD in treating pain has been ongoing since ancient times. Countries from Asia, Europe, and America have used Cannabis as an analgesic.

Prevent Obesity and Diabetes

Once CBD is introduced in the body it will help convert the white fat into brown fat. Brown fat is considered weight reducing as it intensifies the production of insulin and sugar metabolism. We all know that sugar is the major culprit when it comes to weight gain.

In 2006, CBD was introduced to laboratory rats to test its healing effect for diabetes. The experiment was successful as it lowered the incidence of diabetes. Another experiment was conducted by an Israeli-American biopharmaceutical company and again proved the CBD successfully treats diabetes.

Over time, around 4,000 subjects have been studied. Statistical results showed that there was a 16% increase in fasting insulin levels, a 17% decrease in insulin resistance, and the presence of more HDL which helps prevent obesity and diabetes.

Reduce the Risk of Cancer

In 2012, an experiment was conducted on laboratory animals. They were injected with carcinogens. Then they were given doses of CBD. The results showed that those animals with CBD doses did not develop cancer cells in the colon.

Some studies have stated that for an optimal effect, CBD must be mixed with THC when treating cancer. To date, experiments are still being done to find the perfect mixture.

Helps Build Strong Bones

Experiments have been conducted to determine if CBD helps build strong bones and35-50% of those treated with CBD showed positive results.

In a human body, there should be 10% new bones and cartilages built every year to prevent bone-related diseases such as osteoporosis and osteoarthritis. When there is something wrong with the bones, enzymes activate and prevent the generation of new bone cells. Upon introduction of CBD in the system, it has proven to block the function of the enzyme that destroys the bone cells thereby allowing the generation of new cells.

Kills Depression and Mood Swings

CBD is also considered an anti-depressant drug. CBD works by intensifying serotonergic and glutamate cortical signaling through a 5-HT1A receptor-dependent mechanism. CBD targets the depression brought by chronic stress.

Treats Sleeping Disorders

A 15 mg CBD edible has an alerting effect on the subject. An experiment with laboratory animals was conducted with two experimental environments: lights on and lights off. The result of the experiment showed that the subjects were more alert with the lights on. It was concluded that CBD helps treat sleepiness in the daytime brought by nighttime insomnia.

"I have found it's taken the edge off life in general. I feel like my moods aren't in extremes anymore. I can function with day to day activities and not be distracted from bad intrusive thoughts." — Reddit member

Chapter 11

<u>Other Uses of CBD</u>

Uses of CBD for Pets

Interestingly, one of the practical uses of CBD is linked to pets. Please bear in mind that this won't get your dogs, cats and other pets hallucinating or hyped.

Let us explore the perks before we consider using it for our pets.

The use of CBD for pets is perceived to be advantageous and some of these advantages include the following:

- Anti-inflammatory. The anti-inflammatory effects of CBD are actually what make it so favorable in terms of medicating a broad range of conditions. It comes with the capability to collaborate with receptors in immune cells.
- CBD collaborates with CB2 receptors that are commonly found within the immune cells. Hence, by stimulating these receptors, CBD becomes capable of inducing a broad array of immune responses including inflammation.
- CBD can aid in minimizing the pain as well as other symptoms of various conditions such as arthritis, irritable bowel disease, MS, and other chronic inflammations.
- Anti-cancer effects slow down the development of tumors. Malignant tumors and cancer are very common in various pets and can be deadly. There is no cure for cancer and medication generally concentrates on abating the development of a tumor while minimizing the pain and other related symptoms.
- CBD is an effective painkiller. Research has revealed that CBD can assist in managing pain. Some studies showed the capability of CBD to transiently halt anandamide absorption which pertains to a chemical that aids in thwarting pain signals in the brain. As a result, the momentary increase in

anandamide can have different effects and one of these is significantly minimizing pain sensations.

- CBD has also been proven an effective antiemetic and can control both vomiting and nausea and, at the same time, stimulate the appetite. As you know, vomiting and nausea are very common to humans and pets. Essentially, CBD activates 5-HT1A receptors which refer to the same receptor that minimizes anxiety. When this receptor is stimulated, CBD could remarkably diminish feelings of nausea and restrain the successive vomiting reflex.

Uses of CBD for Self-Care or Beauty Products

During the summer, our skin is most likely to be more exposed to the sun. While this is deemed as the perfect time to enjoy lots of adventures, being exposed to too much sunlight can be potentially harmful to the skin. Are you aware that CBD has seized the skincare and beauty market?

Cannabidiol beauty products are not merely used to treat anxiety and various sorts of pain but these are also loaded with anti-inflammatory and antioxidant properties.

The reason why many people fear sun exposure is because UV rays speed up the process of aging. Fortunately, CBD helps slow down aging by acting as a strong defense against skin damage and it also does a wonderful job at promoting collagen production.

In what ways can CBD help maintain good skin?

- A lot of self-care products, such as essential oils, lotions, bath products, skin and beauty products become more effective when combined with cannabidiol. It has been revealed that skincare and beauty products that contain CBD can help with inflammatory skin conditions and other sorts of pain.

- Besides topical products like salves as well as lotions, cannabidiol products that you hold under your tongue, ingest, or inhale have been proven to help a person relax.
- CBD helps relieve various types of pain and aches. Such CBD products are easy to use. A muscle cream that contains CBD helps to relieve sore muscles. You only need to massage it into the aching area and you can instantly feel its soothing effect.
- Bath bombs that contain CBD help encourage relaxation, allow calming sleep, and soothe the skin. They also assist in relieving pain.
- Cannabidiol-infused makeup is broadly acknowledged for its clarifying and soothing effects. This is highly recommended for anyone who is suffering from problems related to eczema and cystic acne. You can apply this serum along with your day and night routine. It is best applied before putting on your makeup.
- There is a lip balm with CBD content. This is especially beneficial during winter seasons. It soothes dry and chapped lips. Even though it is precisely made for the lips, it can also treat your hands, face, and other affected areas of your skin.

The use of CBD is not solely focused on treating anxiety, different types of ailments, and for treating pets. This can also be used if you are suffering from different skin concerns. It can help slow down aging and help improve troubled areas in the skin and other parts of the body.

"I have don't have trouble sleeping, my out of control eating has stopped!

I'm not afraid to speak my mind, if something is bothering me at work, I hesitate less.

I swear I'm in more touch with other people's feelings and my own. I am more mindful to my work and make less mistakes."

– Reddit member

Chapter 12

Sample CBD Recipes

Since CBD has been proven to be adept at providing plenty of health benefits; many health enthusiasts and experts have developed different sumptuous recipes that contain cannabinoids. Here are a few recipes that are easy to make, certified delectable, and can provide several health perks.

RECIPE 1: Burnt Carrots with Cannabidiol Brown Butter

Ingredients:

3 tablespoons of butter (unsalted)
1 tablespoon of extra-virgin olive oil
½ teaspoon of CBD oil
1 6" square sheet of Nori, (torn into bite-size pieces)
Kosher salt
1 pound of big carrots; cut into ½"-thick rounds
1 small garlic clove (crushed)
Flaky sea salt
2 small shallots (cut into ¼" rings)
2 tablespoons of fresh lime juice

Procedure:

1) Put a rack in the top third of oven, and pre-heat to 450-degrees. Stir the olive oil and carrots in a big rimmed baking sheet. Add a pinch of Kosher salt. The carrots must be roasted till slightly burned around the edges and a little tender in the middle. This takes about 17 minutes. Allow mixture to cool.

2) Cook the garlic, Nori, shallots, and butter using a small pan over moderate heat. Stir till butter becomes browned and shallots are brown. Roughly 7 minutes.

3) Add the cannabinoids oil and add the carrots. Carefully stir to combine all ingredients. Season with a pinch of sea salt and drizzle with lime juice.

RECIPE 2: Cannabidiols-infused Parmesan Mashed Potatoes

If you would like to add a slight twist to your regular mashed potato recipe, then you should try this one!

Ingredients:

¼ cup of parmesan cheese (original Parmigiano Reggiano is preferable)
8 cups of pre-prepared mashed potatoes
¼ cup of whipping cream
2 tablespoons of unsalted butter
0.16g Cannabinoids isolate powder
2 teaspoons of salt
2 teaspoons of pepper

Procedure:

1) Mix the whipping cream, mashed potatoes, butter, salt, Cannabinoids isolate powder, parmesan cheese and pepper using the bowl of a stand mixer.

2) Carefully whip all these ingredients until pureed.

3) Move the potato puree to a moderately-sized casserole dish that has been sprayed with a non-stick spray.

4) Top the mashed potatoes with parmesan cheese and then bake at 400F.

5) Let the potatoes cool slightly before serving.

RECIPE 3: Pumpkin Spice Latte Loaf with CBD Icing

Are you allergic to nuts or seeds? Then, start making this CBD-infused recipe!

Ingredients:

For the loaf:
4 medium-sized eggs
1 teaspoon of pumpkin pie spice
1 tablespoon of apple cider
½ cup yuca-root flour
1 teaspoon of baking soda
1 teaspoon of espresso powder
1 cup pumpkin puree

For the Cannabinoids sugarless icing:
¼ cup of coconut butter
1 tablespoon of Cannabinoids coconut oil

Procedure:

1) Pre-heat the oven to 350F.

2) In a bowl, carefully mix the baking soda with apple cider and allow the mixture to fizz. Using a stand mixer, stir in the eggs till peaks form.

3) Combine all the other remaining ingredients until well-mixed.

4) Line a bread loaf pan with parchment paper and carefully pour the batter into the pan.

5) Bake this for half an hour. Put the loaf in a freezer for about half an hour to allow it to cool.

Procedure for the icing:

On low heat, melt the coconut butter with cannabinoids coconut oil till mixed and carefully pour it over the loaf.

"I went to the mall after taking the CBD and my SO said he has never seen me so still before. He said normally I looks like I carry so much weight in my shoulders and he said it was good to see me so calm." – Reddit member

Chapter 13

CBD Case Studies

In this chapter, we will discuss some of the case studies conducted by experts to prove how effective CBD is in treating or alleviating symptoms of certain diseases. The case studies that will be included here are explained simply.

Case Study # 1

Objective: To prove that CBD decreases the onset of seizures or epilepsy attacks of patients suffering from Dravet syndrome (DS) and Lennox-Gastaut syndrome (LGS).

Subject: 15 children and 2 adults with LGS and 7 children with DS

Procedure:

- Subjects were placed on placebo medication for 12 weeks
- After 12 weeks, they were given a medication composed of 98% CBD with a very small amount of THC

Result: Seizures reduced by 39%. Because of this successful study, FDA approved Epidiolex, the first CBD-based drug to manage epilepsy attacks.

Case Study # 2

Objective: To check the impact of CBD on dogs diagnosed with Idiopathic Epilepsy

Subject: 26 client-owned dogs with intractable idiopathic epilepsy

Procedure:

- Dogs were grouped into CBD and placebo group
- The CBD group received CBD-infused oil (2.5 mg/kg [1.1 mg/lb], PO) twice daily for 12 weeks in addition to existing antiepileptic treatments

- The placebo group received non-infused oil under the same conditions

Result: Seizures reduced by 33% in dogs from the CBD group. However, a deeper analysis by another study must be done because the 33% reduction in seizures was manifested only by >/=50% of the dogs from the CBD group. The next experiment will introduce a higher dosage of CBD to the subjects.

Case Study # 3

Objective: To prove that Oral CBD prevents Allodynia and Neurological Dysfunctions to those with Mild Traumatic Brain Injury (TBI)

Subject: Mice with Mild TBI

Procedure:

- 10% of CBD oil was injected into the mice
- After showing adverse effects, Oral CBD was introduced to the mice

Result: Upon injection of CBD oil, the mice developed a chronic pain followed by depression-like symptoms and a decrease in social interaction. After the introduction of oral CBD, the symptoms were reversed and the mice showed improved condition.

Case Study # 4

Objective: To prove that CBD oil can ease the tension felt by patients suffering from Inflammatory Bowel Disease (IBD)

Subject: 82 patients, combined young and adult with IBD

Procedure:

- Administer CBD oil to 15 patients sublingually

- 6 patients were administered with pure CBD oil
- 9 patients were administered with CBD:THC ratio

Results: Improved condition, increase in appetite, lessened pain

Case Study # 5

Objective: To prove that CBD improves the condition of patients with ASD or autism

Subject: 188 ASD patients monitored between the years of 2015 and 2017

Procedure:

Patients were administered with CBD oil containing 30% CBD and 1.5% THC

Results: After 6 months, only 155 patients continued with the treatment; 60% or 93 patients were assessed. From the 93, 28 showed significant improvement, 50 showed moderate improvement, 6 showed slight improvement, and 8 showed no changes at all. The symptom improved was restlessness.

Case Study # 6

Objective: To prove the efficacy of CBD oil to dogs diagnosed with Osteoarthritic pain (OA)

Subject: Dogs with OA

Procedure:

- 2-8 mg of CBD oil and placebo medicine was administered to dogs every 12 hours within 2-4 weeks

Results: Pain was reduced in dogs receiving CBD oil. The assessment showed that 2mg of CBD oil twice a day will alleviate the pain of dogs with OA.

Case Study # 7

Objective: To assess the effect of chronic exposure to CBD to the reproductive function of Swiss male mice

Subject: 12 day-old Swiss male mice

Procedure:

- 1 group were administered with 15 mg CBD
- 1 group were administered with 30 mg CBD
- 1 group were administered with placebo
- The observation lasted 34 days

Results: Sperm abnormalities, impaired sexual activity, the reduced fertility rate

Case Study # 8

Objective: To assess the efficacy of CBD in pain management of patients with cancer

Subject: Series of tests were conducted to cancer patients between the years 1975 and 2017

Procedure:

- Patients were given 2.7-43.2 mg/day THC and 0-40 mg/day CBD

Results: Varying results; some showed improved condition when higher doses of THC were administered, some showed significant improvement with low THC and high CBD doses. However, side effects, such as drowsiness, mental clouding, hypotension, nausea, and vomiting were noted. A further study must still be conducted to prove its efficacy in pain management since only a few patients were part of the initial studies.

Case Study # 9

Objective: To prove the impact of CBD oil on Metastatic Low-Grade Serous Ovarian Carcinoma (LGSOC)

Subject: 81-year-old woman

Procedure:

- The 81-year-old woman who opted to undergo Complimentary Alternative Medicine (CAM) and be treated with CBD Oil for her LGSOC. She opted for this treatment for quality of life. Every month, tests were done like measurements of her CA-125 level.

Results: She was diagnosed with LGSOC in March 2017. In May 2017, she started her CAM with CBD oil treatment. Month on month improvement of her condition was observed. In December 2018, she was totally asymptomatic.

Case Study # 10

Objective: To assess the impact of CBD to treat Anxiety and Sleep Disorders

Subject: 103 patients from a psychiatric ward

Procedure:

- Administer CBD to patients for a few months

Results: Anxiety decreased in 57 patients during the first month of treatment and 48 patients reported sleep patterns improved during the first month of treatment.

Conclusion

We now know that CBD is not dangerous and not even addictive. Surprisingly, a lot of uses have been discovered and proven effective. This paved the way for people to explore and experiment with how CBD will be introduced to the market and the increase of many CBD-based products available.

There is so much information about CBD. At this time, a lot of people, especially in developed countries, accept the efficacy of CBD in treating illnesses. The question now is how it will be institutionalized. There seems to be a lack of information dissemination about the positive sides of CBD. That is why books like this are being written and distributed to increase awareness.

While debates are ongoing on how to institutionalize the use of CBD, we hope that this book gave you so many insights. May this book increased your awareness and perhaps create that interest to try CBD in treating illnesses identified in the narrative of this book.

It's a huge advantage that our generation is discovering that CBD is the answer to some illnesses. May in this generation also witness how this substance will be legally accepted.

It is comforting to know that critical illnesses such as cancer can now be cured or alleviated and many diseases can now be prevented. More will be discovered about this wonder plant Cannabis. As the saying goes, everything here on Earth has a purpose.

References/Links

https://myhealthmonster.com/cbd-studies/
https://www.reddit.com/r/CBD/
http://www.pdfonlinereader.com/WebPdf2/index.html
http://www.pdfonlinereader.com/WebPdf2/editor.html
https://www.cannabiscompliancefirm.com/news/2018/4/25/the-cannabis-plant-the-difference-between-hemp-and-marijuana
https://www.livescience.com/63452-what-is-cannabis-oil.html
https://www.prima.co/magazine/top-4-hemp-myths-debunked
https://www.americanspa.com/cbd/debunking-myths-about-cbd
https://floydsofleadville.com/debunking-3-common-misconceptions-about-cbd/
https://www.healthline.com/health/myths-about-cbd#2
https://pubchem.ncbi.nlm.nih.gov/compound/Cannabidiol
https://www.worldofmolecules.com/drugs/cannabidiol-molecule.html
https://adai.uw.edu/marijuana/factsheets/cannabinoids.htm
https://canrelieve.com/learn-about-cbd/cbd-dosage/
https://www.healthline.com/health/your-cbd-guide#dosage
https://bigskybotanicals.com/blog/cbd-product-types-guide/
https://www.verywellhealth.com/cbd-oil-benefits-uses-side-effects-4174562
https://www.webmd.com/vitamins/ai/ingredientmono-1439/cannabidiol-cbd
https://www.mayoclinic.org/healthy-lifestyle/consumer-health/expert-answers/is-cbd-safe-and-effective/faq-20446700
https://usa.inquirer.net/33919/warning-cbd-users-must-read-this
https://www.webmd.com/pain-management/news/20180507/cbd-oil-all-the-rage-but-is-it-safe-effective#3
https://www.medicalnewstoday.com/articles/317221.php

https://www.healthline.com/health/how-to-take-cbd#what-to-look-for
https://www.healthline.com/health/cbd-dosage
https://www.cbdoil.org/cbd-dosage-guide/
https://restartcbd.com/cbd-dosing-charts/
https://www.tuck.com/cbd-dosage/
https://www.healthline.com/health/cbd-dosage#takeaway
https://www.thegrowthop.com/cannabis-culture/what-is-the-best-time-of-day-to-take-cbd
https://www.needlerockcbd.com/best-time-of-the-day-to-take-cbd-oil/
https://cbdoilusers.com/best-time-of-day-to-take-cbd-oil/
https://www.royalqueenseeds.com/blog-when-and-how-often-should-you-take-cbd-n1071
https://echoconnection.org/whens-best-time-take-cbd/
https://www.healthline.com/health/how-to-take-cbd#what-to-look-for
https://www.anaviimarket.com/blogs/news/what-to-look-for-when-buying-cbd-oil
https://medium.com/cbd-origin/10-things-to-know-before-you-buy-cbd-online-or-anywhere-really-db9813f32884
https://joyorganics.com/10-tips-for-choosing-quality-cbd-products/
https://cbdoilreview.org/cbd-cannabidiol/cbd-oil-product-buying-tips/
https://www.petmd.com/dog/general-health/cannabis-oil-dogs-everything-you-need-know
https://www.akc.org/expert-advice/health/cbd-oil-dogs/
https://cannabissupplementsforpets.com/benefits-of-cbd-for-dogs/
https://www.self.com/story/cbd-skin-care
https://www.bhg.com/news/guide-to-cbd-self-care/
https://fashionlifemag.com/2019/05/29/a-full-guide-to-cbd-beauty-self-care-products/

https://www.bonappetit.com/recipe/burnt-carrots-with-cbd-brown-butter
https://royalcbd.com/cbd-oil-recipes/
https://www.consciouslifestylemag.com/cbd-health-benefits/
https://www.verywellhealth.com/cbd-oil-benefits-uses-side-effects-4174562
https://www.health.harvard.edu/blog/cannabidiol-cbd-what-we-know-and-what-we-dont-2018082414476
https://www.webmd.com/vitamins/ai/ingredientmono-1439/cannabidiol-cbd
https://www.healthline.com/nutrition/cbd-oil-benefits#section7